Dr. Earl Mindell's

What You Should
Know About
Natural Health For Men

Dr. Earl Mindell's

What You Should Know About Natural Health For Men

Earl L. Mindell, R.Ph., Ph.D.

with Virginia L. Hopkins

Keats Publishing, Inc.   New Canaan, Connecticut

Dr. Earl Mindell's What You Should Know About Natural Health For Men is intended solely for informational and educational purposes, and not as medical advice. Please consult a medical or health professional if you have questions about your health.

Library of Congress Cataloging-in-Publication Data

Mindell, Earl.
  [What you should know about natural health for men]
  Dr. Earl Mindell's What you should know about natural health for men / by Earl Mindell, with Virginia L. Hopkins.
      p.   cm.
  Includes bibliographical references and index.
  ISBN 0-87983-753-5
  1. Prostate—Diseases—Prevention. 2. Impotence—Prevention. 3. Men—Health and hygiene. 4. Naturopathy.
I. Hopkins, Virginia. II. Title.
RC889.M555   1996
616.6'5—dc20   96-11244
                                                      CIP

Printed in the United States of America

Keats Publishing, Inc.
27 Pine Street (Box 876)
New Canaan, Connecticut 06840-0876

98 97 96   6 5 4 3 2 1

Contents

We would like to thank Maria Gordon for her expert assistance in writing and researching this book.

PART I:
How to Stay Sexually Healthy

CHAPTER 1

Getting Reacquainted With the Male Anatomy

With his best-selling book, *Men Are from Mars, Women Are from Venus,* author John Gray created a new vocabulary of male-female relationships based on explaining the differences between the sexes. While some of these differences are based on environment and cultural values, most of them are based on the biological facts of anatomy and hormones. Although as human beings the sexes are more alike than different, men do have unique physical attributes, challenges and concerns.

TESTOSTERONE: THE MALE HORMONE

Testosterone is the hormone that transforms a boy into a man. Men produce ten times more testosterone in their bodies than women do. Most of it is produced in the testes, but some is also produced in the adrenal glands.

Testosterone levels in a male during fetal development in the womb are higher than they are from shortly after birth until puberty. When the fetus is only four weeks old, testosterone begins to stimulate the growth of the penis, testes, scrotum and prostate gland, and suppress the growth of female characteristics. Testosterone also causes the testes to descend into the scrotum.

When a boy reaches puberty, increased levels of testosterone will cause his penis and scrotum to enlarge by eight to ten times, his voice will become deeper, his skin will become thicker, the amount of hair on his body will increase, and his muscles will become better defined. Testosterone is also responsible for male pattern baldness, and men's tendency to be more aggressive than women.

THE TESTES: THE MALE REPRODUCTIVE ORGAN

The testes in the man are essentially the same organs as the ovaries in the woman. In fact, if you look at an anatomical drawing, they appear nearly identical in outer shape except that the ovaries sit up in the abdomen and the testes hang down between the legs in a sac called the scrotum. However, a key difference is that the ovaries produce relatively large amounts of estrogen and progesterone, while the testes produce relatively large amounts of testosterone.

The testes have two jobs to do in the male body. One job is to participate in the production of sperm, and the other is to secrete hormones into the bloodstream. If there is a deficiency of testosterone, or an excess of estrogen, the testes may not descend. Some ten percent of boys are born with an undescended testicle, but 97 percent of them descend within a few weeks of birth. Of those that don't descend in infancy, the vast majority descend under the influence of increased testosterone at puberty. An undescended testicle will produce hormones, but it won't produce viable sperm. A testicle that doesn't descend by about the age of five usually won't be able to produce live sperm.

The testes rest in a loose sac of skin called the scrotal sac. There is a good biological reason for the testes to be located outside the body: sperm develop better in temperatures lower than body temperature. If the temperature drops too much, special muscles pull the testes back up into the body. If it goes too high, they drop more.

Men who are concerned about their fertility should wear all-cotton boxer shorts and avoid hot baths to keep from overheating the testes.

XENOESTROGENS AND THEIR EFFECT ON MEN

Since boys produce minimal amounts of testosterone, the presence of an undescended testicle after infancy would suggest the presence of excess estrogen.

Some herbalists recommend saw palmetto berry for boys with an undescended testicle, to enhance the activity of the small amount of testosterone present in a young boy.

I strongly recommend that boys with an undescended testicle avoid environmental estrogens, known as "xenoestrogens," as much as possible. Pervasive petrochemical pollution has dropped us all into a sea of xenoestrogens, and the long term consequences for men are devastating. The rate of undescended testicles in boys has doubled since the end of World War II, when petrochemical products and byproducts, including pesticides, plastics and air pollution, were introduced into our environment. During that same period, men's sperm count has dropped by half, with a corresponding rise in infertility. Some studies indicate that an undescended testicle has a much higher risk of becoming cancerous in adulthood.

Testicular cancer, which tends to strike men between the ages of 35 and 50, and is the most common type of cancer among men aged 15 to 35, has quadrupled since the 1940s. Biopsies done on testicular tumors in children show the presence of abnormal fetal-like cells, suggesting that whatever went awry had its source in the womb. Studies of reproductive abnormalities in animals such as seagulls demonstrate that exposure to excessive estrogen in the womb causes reproductive abnormalities in the offspring. While the predisposition to testicular cancer may be genetic, or begin in the womb, living a healthy lifestyle and avoiding xenoestrogens is the best preventive strategy men can employ.

HOW TO AVOID XENOESTROGENS

While no one source of normal exposure to xenoestrogens is likely to cause estrogen excess, it has a cumulative effect, as we are exposed to it in many small doses. Avoiding xenoestrogens involves avoiding all meat and fowl unless you know for sure it is "organic," meaning raised without hormones. Nearly all livestock raised for eating in the United States is given estrogen-like substances to increase fat content.

Pesticides, herbicides and fungicides, which can act as potent xenoestrogens in the body in very small amounts, must also be avoided. This means no lawn or garden sprays, no bug sprays or flea bombs of any kind, and organically grown—without the customary application of pesticides or artificial fertilizers—fruits and vegetables.

Many soaps, including laundry soaps and dish soaps, contain substances called nonylphenols, which are surfactants that also act as potent xenoestrogens. I recommend that you look in your health food store for environmentally friendly "green" products without nonylphenols.

Many types of plastic shed xenoestrogens, so avoid heating food or cooking in plastic.

At the same time, it's important to eat vegetables, which contain "phytoestrogens." This type of plant estrogen will take up estrogen receptors in the body, effectively blocking the action of the real thing.

SPERM AND SEMEN

Sperm is manufactured in the testes, but it doesn't leave the body directly from there. First it makes its way to the epididymis, a long tube attached to the back of each testicle, where it picks up a tail, enabling it to swim. Then it moves on to another tube called the vas deferens, where it travels up into the groin, behind the bladder and into the prostate. The sperm are stored in the end of the vas deferens until they enter the urethra at the time of ejaculation. On their journey from the vas deferens to the penis, sperm are mixed with various fluids from the prostate and the seminal vesicles. This fluid protects the sperm, makes them swim faster and harder, and makes the vagina more receptive. This mixture is called semen, or ejaculate. Semen is made up of fructose, glucose, citric acid, zinc, selenium, vitamin E, proteins and enzymes.

Although sperm make up an extremely tiny percentage of ejaculate, just 3 percent, there are an average of 400 million sperm in one batch of semen. Only a few will make it all the way to the waiting egg, which is gigantic in size compared to the sperm, and only one sperm will actually penetrate the egg and cause conception.

Because the prostate gland can be the cause of so many problems as men age, Part II of this book is devoted to it.

THE URETHRA

The tube descending from the bladder and out to the end of penis, which carries urine and semen, is called the urethra. On its way to the penis, the urethra passes through the prostate gland, where it picks up fluids for semen during ejaculation. During ejaculation a muscle in the urethra clamps down, blocking urine from the passageway. This also keeps semen headed down into the penis instead of back toward the bladder. You will hear a lot more about the urethra in the section on the prostate.

THE PENIS

The penis is made of three cylindrical spongelike bodies that contain blood, the urethra, and the head, or glans, at the end. When the penis is erect, the spongelike bodies are engorged with blood and the veins that carry blood out of the penis are constricted. The process of erection is under the involuntary control of the autonomic nervous system, and can be brought about by psychological or physical stimuli. Interestingly, the penis can become erect through psychological stimulation alone, such as a daydream, or physical stimulation alone, such as masturbation. The glans is the part of penis most sensitive to stimulation.

The average penis is about 3.5 inches long flaccid, and 5 inches long erect, representing a 300 percent increase in volume! Men get an average of 5 erections a night. Contrary to popular notion, penis size doesn't vary much and has little to do with how large or tall a man is. Penis length *is* affected by obesity—fat around the waist can, in effect, absorb the end of the penis, making it shorter.

CHAPTER 2

How to Prevent Impotence

Impotence, or the inability to attain or maintain an erection, can be caused ·by either psychological or physical factors. Researchers estimate that some 25 percent of men over the age of 50 suffer from some form of impotence, also called erectile dysfunction. In older men, the cause of impotence is nearly always of physical origin.

There is something to be said for the axiom, "Use it or lose it," when it comes to sexual function. Having regular sex may be one of the best deterrents to impotence. It stimulates circulation, hormones and seminal secretions, and brings energy to the genital area. Not to mention the fact that it's fun, feels good, can be good exercise and, perhaps most important, is an opportunity for closeness and intimacy with a loved one, an important factor in good health. Masturbation certainly doesn't have all the benefits of having sex with another person, but can be an important outlet when a sexual partner isn't available.

The four major physical causes of impotence are alcohol, cigarette smoking, prescription drugs and the types of heart disease that produce clogged blood vessels. Other causes include poor diet—especially too much sugar—diabetes, hypothyroidism (low thyroid), excess estrogen, stress and depression.

According to research done at the Boston University School of Medicine, men who have heart disease, diabetes, or high blood pressure have four times the risk of becoming impotent as they age as men who are free of these chronic diseases.

ALCOHOL

Alcohol interferes with many parts of the body related to sexual performance, and excessive alcohol use will actually shrink the testicles and lower your production of testosterone. Men who are under the influence of alcohol often think they are better lovers because their inhibitions are lowered, but their erections tend to be significantly softer, their coordination compromised and their reflexes slower. Shakespeare probably said it best in Macbeth when he described alcohol as that which "provokes the desire, but . . . takes away the performance." Alcohol is also a vitamin robber, a fact which can interfere with sexual performance over the long term.

CIGARETTES

Cigarettes interfere with sex drive and with erections via many mechanisms, including clogged blood vessels, poor physical condition, and poisoning from the wide array of toxins present in tobacco (most of these toxins are added by the tobacco companies, by the way). The nicotine in tobacco acts to constrict your blood vessels. Every cigarette smoked means less blood will reach the penis when it is stimulated. The Boston University research on impotence showed that even after being treated for heart disease, men who continued smoking had a 56 percent higher risk of becoming impotent, while those who didn't smoke only had a 21 percent risk. Men who quit smoking generally notice they have firmer erections after just a few weeks.

PRESCRIPTION DRUGS

Many, many prescription drugs, particularly those prescribed for older men, can cause impotence. The vast majority of men should be able to remain sexually vigorous well into their eighties. My guess is that the myth that sex drive drops around the age of 50 has more to do with the drugs doctors start handing out at that age rather than any real physical incapability. This is one of the best reasons I can think of to live healthily and avoid prescription drugs if at all possible. Chronic problems such as high blood pressure and high cholesterol can almost always be solved with a healthy lifestyle and some nutritional and herbal supplements. Nearly every heart disease drug has a natural counterpart that doesn't cause side effects. Only a tiny percentage of men ever need to suffer from impotence due to prescription drugs.

If you're suffering from impotence and are taking a prescription drug, call your pharmacist or your doctor and ask if one of the side effects of the drug is impotence. Combining one or more drugs can also cause unreported side effects, including impotence. If you're taking more than one drug, including over-the-counter drugs, it could be causing your impotence, even if that is not listed as a side effect.

Some Common Types of Drugs That Can Cause Impotence

- Antibiotics
- Antihistamines (for allergies and sinus congestion)
- Anticholinergics (used for ulcers and other gastrointestinal disorders, to suppress nausea, for

tremors caused by Parkinson's disease and psychiatric drugs, sometimes for asthma)

- Anticonvulsants
- Antidepressants
- Antihypertensives (drugs that lower blood pressure)
- Antipsychotics
- H2 blockers such as Tagamet, Pepcid and Zantac
- Sedatives and tranquilizers
- Many of the drugs used to treat heart disease, including beta blockers, calcium channel blockers, ace inhibitors and antiangina drugs
- Painkillers such as indomethacin, naproxen and naltrexone

CLOGGED ARTERIES

Clogged arteries are the leading cause of death in the United States, and they may also be the leading cause of impotence. Think about it. The physical mechanism of erection is dependent upon blood flow. The arteries around your heart aren't the only ones that become clogged when you have heart disease. The arteries in your penis are suffering the same fate. In fact, impotence can be one of the first outward signs of clogged arteries.

Contrary to what mainstream medical doctors would have you believe, clogged arteries (and most types of heart disease for that matter) *are* reversible through good nutrition and a healthy lifestyle. This has been conclusively proven by Dr. Dean Ornish, who put his heart disease patients on an intensive heart-healthy lifestyle and got excellent results.

America's poor diet contributes heavily to its rate of heart disease. We eat too much fat, too many processed foods, and not enough fresh vegetables. In the

1950s, the Japanese diet was 16 percent fat, and they had almost no incidence of heart disease. Today their diet is 26 percent fat, and heart disease is the second leading cause of death in Japan. In the U.S. the average diet contains 36 to 40 percent fat.

Worldwide, cultures eating less meat and more fish, fruits and vegetables, and drinking more wine, have significantly lower rates of death from heart disease. Furthermore, there is a strong correlation between diets high in polyunsaturated fatty acids (vegetable oils prone to oxidation/rancidity) and a high rate of death from heart disease, and correspondingly lower death rates in those cultures that consume more monounsaturated fats such as olive oil.

Those countries with the highest intake of antioxidants and bioflavonoids have the lowest death rates from heart disease, with Japan having a much higher intake and a much lower rate of death than any of the other countries.

In the next chapter I will go into detail about how you can follow a lifestyle that will help you have a long and active sex life.

POOR DIET

A poor diet doesn't just clog your arteries, it also robs you of important vitamins, depletes cells of oxygen and energy, and creates blood sugar imbalances. One of your keys to a physically healthy sex life is good circulation, and a good diet and exercise are your keys to good circulation. I'll talk about how to maximize your sex life by maximizing your diet in detail in the next chapter.

Men who have low HDL or "good" cholesterol have a much greater risk of being impotent than those who have normal or high HDL cholesterol. You can raise

your HDL cholesterol by following the program I'll
give you in the next chapter.

DIABETES

Diabetes afflicts millions of Americans, and impotence
is one of the most distressing side effects of this disease. The most tragic part of this scenario is that
nearly all adult-onset diabetes can be prevented and
even reversed if caught early enough, with diet and
lifestyle.

Because diabetes medication theoretically has to be
taken every day for the rest of your life, it's a huge
business that generates big bucks. That's why you
don't hear much about people who beat diabetes by
changing their lifestyle. And it's much easier for a
doctor to prescribe a daily shot or pill to control your
diabetes than it is for him or her to encourage you to
lose weight, exercise and start eating a nutritious diet.
More than 90 percent of the diabetes in the U.S. is
caused by obesity, poor diet and lack of exercise. All
of these causes are under your control, and it's a lot
easier to prevent diabetes than it is to treat it once
you have it.

In countries where people eat a diet low in fat and
sugar and high in whole foods such as unrefined
grains and fresh fruits and vegetables, diabetes is almost nonexistent.

Most mainstream doctors are unable to help their
patients control their diabetes naturally because they
don't understand the basics of nutrition. They recommend a high-carbohydrate diet that avoids sugar, but
they fail to distinguish between refined carbohydrates
and complex carbohydrates! If you eat pancakes,
bread or baked goods made from white flour, your
blood sugar will rise almost as fast as it would if you
just ate white sugar. It's important for diabetics to eat

unrefined carbohydrates such as whole-grain bread, brown rice and beans. If you have a hard time digesting whole grains, introduce them to your diet gradually, and eat them in small amounts. You don't need a lot of carbohydrates to stay healthy—what's most important is the *quality* of your carbohydrates.

I find it fascinating that the very nutrients that are stripped out of refined carbohydrates—chromium, zinc, manganese and vanadium—are the same ones that are critical to maintaining stable blood sugar, and are also the very ones that diabetics have been found to be deficient in. If you are at risk for diabetes, or have adult-onset diabetes, the major focus of your diet should be fresh vegetables, legumes (such as beans and soy products) and nuts, followed by lean protein, unrefined carbohydrates and small amounts of fresh fruits. Refined carbohydrates and sugar should not ever be consumed if you are at risk for diabetes or have it. That may sound tough, but isn't it tougher to suffer from the effects of diabetes, which include heart disease, blindness and numbness in the extremities?

While it may not be possible for many diabetics to get completely off insulin, you can dramatically reduce your need for insulin by taking the following supplements. Be sure to work with a health-care professional who can help you monitor your progress.

Chromium picolinate works hand in hand with insulin to stabilize blood sugar. Take 200 to 600 mcg daily.

Vanadyl sulfate (a form of vanadium). Start at 6 mg and increase the dose until you get results, up to 100 mg daily. You can use this trace mineral, with chromium, to stabilize your blood sugar. At high doses vanadyl can cause cramping and diarrhea—back off the dose if that happens, and don't use high doses for more than three weeks. Don't use vanadyl sulfate if you are hypoglycemic.

Zinc will help your body use insulin more efficiently.

Be sure you're getting 15 mg daily. Most multivitamins contain this amount.

Manganese plays an important role in regulating blood sugar. You should be getting 2 to 5 mg daily. Check your multivitamin.

Onions and garlic can also help lower blood sugar naturally and should be a regular part of the diet of a diabetic. Other herbs and foods that can help lower blood sugar include fenugreek seeds, ginseng, fresh berries, fish, soybeans, fresh vegetables, and cinnamon.

Foods that raise blood sugar include refined sugar, refined grains, carrots, potatoes, processed cereals, raisins, pasta, yams and oranges.

Another key to maintaining stable blood sugar and beating diabetes is keeping your weight down and getting plenty of exercise.

Your need for insulin can drop quickly if you follow my advice, and the less insulin you need, the less chance you'll suffer from the effects of diabetes. I can't stress enough that, if you have diabetes, it is important to work with a health-care professional who can help you monitor your blood sugar carefully as you take these steps. This program does work!

HYPOTHYROIDISM

The thyroid gland is one of your body's central command posts for regulating metabolism, the rate at which you generate energy in your body. Hypothyroidism is a deficiency in the production of thyroid hormones by the thyroid gland. It is more common in women than men, but when it afflicts men one of its side effects can be a decrease in sex drive. Other symptoms of hypothyroidism are weakness, slow speech, cold hands and feet, unexplained gain in weight and difficulty losing it, fatigue, dry skin and headaches.

Blood tests that check your thyroid levels may not accurately diagnose mild hypothyroidism. One of the best ways to find out whether your thyroid gland is up to par is to take your basal body temperature. This is your body temperature upon waking, before doing anything else, even sitting up. You take your basal body temperature by putting the thermometer under your armpit. Your basal body temperature should be between 97.8 and 98.2 degrees Fahrenheit.

If your temperature is low and you suspect you may have hypothyroidism, the first thing to do is find out whether you're getting enough iodine in your diet. You only need very small amounts of iodine, 1 mg daily, but not getting it can seriously impact the functioning of your thyroid gland. Table salt that you buy in the supermarket has iodine in it, and if your salt consumption is normal you should be getting plenty of iodine in your daily diet. If you're on a heavily salt-restricted diet, you may not be getting enough iodine. Seafood is the best source of iodine.

Another way to boost your thyroid gland is to buy a desiccated thyroid supplement, which you can find at most health food stores. This may be enough to boost you out of a mild thyroid deficiency. If that doesn't help and you still suspect a thyroid deficiency, see a doctor for a prescription thyroid supplement.

EXCESS ESTROGEN

As I mentioned earlier, petrochemical pollution has dropped us all into a sea of synthetic chemicals that behave like estrogen, known as xenoestrogens. No one source of xenoestrogens is going to cause a man to grow breasts or show other signs of feminization, but the effects are cumulative and have an especially potent effect on the fetus.

I believe that the steadily rising rate of prostate enlargement, prostate cancer, testicular cancer and infertility among men is due to chronic long-term exposure to xenoestrogens through meat, pesticides, plastic residues and surfactants in soaps. One group of researchers in England even found that the estrogens excreted in the urine of women taking birth control pills were making their way intact through sewage treatment plants and into the food chain. Remember, estrogen is the female hormone, and its presence will actually oppose testosterone, in effect reducing testosterone levels.

Let's review the steps you can take to reduce your exposure to xenoestrogens:

Avoid all meat and fowl unless you know for sure it is "organic," meaning raised without hormones. Nearly all livestock raised for eating in the United States is given estrogen-like substances to increase fat content.

Avoid pesticides, herbicides and fungicides, which can act as potent xenoestrogens in the body in very small amounts. This means no lawn or garden sprays, no bug sprays or flea bombs of any kind, and organic fruits and vegetables.

Avoid exposure to laundry soaps and dish soaps which contain substances called nonylphenols, which are surfactants that also act as potent xenoestrogens. In the first chapter I recommended using environmentally friendly, nonylphenol-free "green" products. Even if you do not have to eat or drink these substances, they are fat-soluble and will enter directly through your skin.

Avoid heating food or cooking in plastic, as many plastics shed.

Eat plenty of fresh, organic vegetables and soy products, which contain "phytoestrogens." This type of plant estrogen will take up estrogen receptors in the body, effectively blocking or reducing the action of the real thing. Soy is my favorite phytoestrogen.

These steps are especially important if you are trying to father a child, and are also important for a woman who is trying to become pregnant or is pregnant. The most significant harm by xenoestrogens is caused by exposure in the womb, where it can cause reproductive abnormalities, particularly in males.

CHAPTER 3

Prescription for a Long and Active Sex Life

Why is it so difficult to change our unhealthy habits? By now you would have to live in a cave on a mountain top not to know that a high-fat diet of junk food is going to take you straight down the royal road to heart disease. Mainstream medicine considers it so difficult to change an unhealthy lifestyle that most doctors will write you a prescription for a drug they know has unpleasant side effects before they will even consider suggesting you lose weight and get some exercise. We could save billions of dollars every year in health-care costs if we just changed our eating habits and our sedentary lifestyles a little bit.

Food is an emotionally charged subject. Our "comfort foods," which we eat when we're upset or stressed, are usually fat-laden, sweet and soft, or salty and crunchy. In other words, what Americans reach for when they want a snack or when they're stressed, which is most of the time, is sugar, white flour, salt and hydrogenated oils. When we eat a meal it often comes out of a can or a box, and is stripped of its nutritional value, with a few token vitamins added back in. To add insult to injury, processed foods contain a veritable chemistry lab of additives, preservatives and dyes, many of which cause allergic reactions.

Combine fatty, sugary, salty snacks and processed nutrition-free foods with little to no exercise, and you have a recipe for chronic illnesses such as arthritis, diabetes and heart disease. Headaches, back pain, fatigue, depression, foggy thinking, memory loss, and high blood pressure are some other common effects of this type of diet. Lack of sex drive and impotence by the age of 60 are frequently the long-term consequences of the typical American lifestyle.

If you begin feeling the debilitating effects of the standard American diet when you're in your fifties, and your life expectancy is 75, that gives you about 25 years of a less-than-optimal life, complete with drugs, surgeries and chronic pain. But there is no reason to suffer that fate! You will be amazed at how dramatically your energy will pick up and how much better you'll feel emotionally and mentally when you start eating whole foods and getting some exercise. I call this a "high-potency" lifestyle!

When you change your lifestyle and start giving up the pastries and potato chips, it's important to do it gradually and to give yourself substitute treats. You can't just yank away your favorite comfort foods and expect to experience success. For example, if you're working to give up sugary desserts after dinner, substitute your favorite sweet fruits, even if they're out of season and expensive. You're worth it, and it will help ease you out of the habit. Please don't use the sugar substitute aspartame; it is a brain excitotoxin that is likely to cause more problems than it will solve.

If you're working to give up potato chips, substitute roasted nuts or seeds (fresh, not rancid, please!), which may be equally high in fat, but will spare you the hydrogenated oils found in snack foods and will add all kinds of good nutrition.

CAN WATER IMPROVE YOUR SEX LIFE?

Water may be the cheapest, easiest way to improve your sex life. Americans are so chronically dehydrated you'd think we lived in a desert and that water was a scarce commodity. In truth, clean water is scarce and we often drink coffee, tea and soft drinks instead of water.

Drinking plenty of clean water is essential to good health. I recommend everyone drink 6 to 8 glasses a day.

And guess what, guys—I know this sounds too simple to be true, but drinking a tall glass of clean water half an hour or so before having sex can make all the difference in your ability to get and maintain an erection. It makes sense, doesn't it? Blood, which is what an erection is made of, is made primarily of water. It's not too likely that if your body is dehydrated it's going to give up some precious water for an erection! It's amazing what staying hydrated can do for your sex life!

SUGAR IS A SEX BUSTER

I can't say enough bad things about sugar. It will do more to diminish (so to speak) your sex life than almost any other food (alcohol and drugs can do more harm, but they aren't foods). While glucose, a form of sugar, is essential to life, what Americans stuff into their bodies by the dozens of pounds every year in the form of white, refined sugar is not only *not* essential to life, it is detrimental to life and to good health.

Your body can make all the sugar it needs from carbohydrates, and we all get plenty of those when we eat grains, legumes, potatoes, rice, corn and other starchy vegetables. The sugar we get from cakes, candies, ice cream, pastries, soft drinks and dozens of other sources will contribute to heart disease, diabetes and arthritis. It will make your capillaries "baggy," and less able to deliver oxygen and other nutrients to your cells. It will run your life because you'll always be looking for your next sugar fix to boost your flagging energy caused by your last sugar fix.

Please don't fall for the advertising gimmick that refined fructose is not as bad a sugar as the others—it may even be worse, because there is evidence that it suppresses the immune system when eaten regularly. Sucrose and malt are also sugars. Regardless of how quickly or slowly your body processes a sugar, it's still a sugar. If you don't burn it off, it will add to your fat.

You can get away with occasional sugar snacks if you're athletic and burning off calories intensively. But if you're not burning off those sugar calories right away, they're not doing you any good. They are devoid of nutrition beyond supplying glucose to brain and muscles (most of us have a more than adequate supply), and any energy benefit they give you will result in lower energy within half an hour to an hour.

I'm not against having a sweet now and then, but most Americans are addicted to sugar. If you're eating foods high in refined sugars more than a few times a week, kicking the sugar habit may be the single best thing you can do for your health.

HYDROGENATED OILS DAMAGE ARTERIES

I'm really down on the hydrogenated oils you'll find in nearly every processed snack food in America. I'm convinced they've contributed heavily to our astronomical rate of death from heart disease. These vegetable oils are chemically processed so that they're partially saturated to keep them from going rancid. They damage your arteries and take up receptor sites for the essential fatty acids so important to good health. These extremely harmful oils have been pushed on the public for years by the very powerful vegetable oil industry, to the great detriment of our national health.

Eating unprocessed vegetable oils isn't the answer either, unless you're pressing them by hand in your home and using them immediately! Vegetable and nut oils (corn, safflower, peanut, soy) are very unstable polyunsaturated oils and go rancid easily. In fact, most vegetable oils are rancid before you even open the bottle, and are certainly well on their way within a few days of exposure to air. Rancid oils smell bad, but even worse, they wreak havoc on your arteries by setting loose more free radicals than any amount of antioxidants can handle, which then damage your arteries. The body attempts to repair this damage with cholesterol, but if you have too much LDL or "bad" cholesterol, the repair job will just act like a magnet for more LDL cholesterol.

Cholesterol in and of itself is not bad for you. In fact, it is necessary to good health. All of your steroid hormones (including testosterone) are made from cholesterol. Cut out too much cholesterol from your diet and you're likely to suffer from a low sex drive, fatigue and depression. Your body manufactures about 75 percent of its own cholesterol, and the remaining 25 percent comes from diet. Any excess cholesterol is simply excreted in a healthy person and does not clog the arteries. What *is* bad for you is oxidized cholesterol, the kind that is created when it meets up with rancid oils and hydrogenated oils, or when you're low on antioxidants.

Your best sources of healthy oil for everyday use are olive oil and canola oil. Olive oil is a stable monounsaturated fat that doesn't go rancid easily and in its unrefined form is packed with nutrition. It can improve "good" HDL cholesterol levels and doesn't break down when used in cooking at low heats. Canola oil is also a monounsaturated oil. While it is processed to remove some harmful ingredients, and is not packed with nutrition like olive oil is, it is a good choice for baking because it doesn't have much flavor and is a light oil.

I don't want you to be scared of saturated fats, either. Saturated fat has been unjustly maligned by the vegetable oil industry. In truth, it's an *excess* of saturated fat that will contribute to heart disease. Moderate amounts of saturated fat are fine, as long as they're combined with plenty of fresh fruits and vegetables and exercise. Moderate means a maximum of one or two small portions (4 ounces) of red meat per week. Don't worry about eating coconut oil or meat, just eat them in small amounts. I like to keep my fat calories to about 25 percent of my calories, and my saturated fat intake is about 10 to 12 percent of that.

Too much fat will beef you up but it won't beef up your sex life. In a study measuring fat consumption and testosterone levels, men who drank a fatty shake watched their testosterone levels drop by thirty percent within four hours.

Essential fatty acids (EFAs), on the other hand, are vital to good health. It's important to get your essential fatty acids by eating fish once or twice a week, and by eating a variety of whole grains, fruits, vegetables and legumes. Most Americans are badly deficient EFAs raising the risk of heart disease and arthritis, because they're eating nutrition-free hydrogenated oils.

As I mentioned earlier, soy is one of my favorite phytoestrogens. I recommend that you incorporate it into your daily diet in place of red meat for many reasons. It is an excellent protein, is packed with nutrition, and contains substances which inhibit cancer and lower cholesterol. You can use soy milk instead of cow's milk, you can eat tofu with just about anything, you can eat miso soup, or you can use tempeh as a meat substitute.

EXERCISE YOUR BODY TO REV UP YOUR SEX LIFE

Having sex takes a lot of energy, and the better shape your body is in, the better shape your sex life will be in. Exercise improves circulation, strengthens the heart and muscles, lowers blood pressure and cholesterol, helps the body rid itself of toxins, increases lung capacity, improves endurance, and will give you an overall feeling of well-being and energy. People who exercise tend to be bright-eyed and bushy-tailed, with a twinkle in the eye and a bounce in the step. Because I travel so much, my favorite form of exercise is brisk walking. I can do it anywhere, and 30 minutes a day four or five times a week keeps me fit and trim. You can ride a bike, weed the garden, rake the lawn, swim, take an aerobics or dance class, or just about anything else that's enjoyable. Any type of moderate exercise that gets your heart going and makes you sweat a little will work fine.

Research supports the exercise-and-better-sex-life connection. In one study, a group of 78 previously sedentary but healthy men (average age 48) jogged or bicycled for an hour a day, 3.5 days per week. A control group of 17 men did not get any regular strenuous or aerobic exercise.

After just nine months the exercise group had a 30 percent increase in the amount of time they had intercourse, with a 26 percent increase in their frequency of orgasms. The control group's rate of intercourse dropped in the same time span.

Chances are, the exercise had a myriad of effects on these men, including an increase in self-esteem. They looked better and felt better, their blood pressure and cholesterol dropped, and they cut their body fat by 19 percent. Speeding up their metabolism with exercise may have also increased their testosterone levels.

Exercise is an excellent stress buster, and stress can put a real damper on your sex life. When you're under chronic stress, your body releases adrenal hormones that over time will throw your body chemistry out of balance. Adrenal hormones are meant for occasional use only—say when a sabertooth tiger is chasing you. When we call on them constantly, with no physical outlet, we're heading for trouble. Exercise is one of the best ways you can neutralize the physical damage stress can do, and it is also a powerful relaxant. However, if you overdo the exercise, it will affect your libido. Moderation is the watchword here.

If exercise isn't enough to de-stress your life, I highly recommend taking classes in one of the Asian movement disciplines such as yoga, chi gong or tai chi, which are easy to find these days nearly everywhere in North America. Learning a form of meditation can also help in coping with stress.

CHAPTER 4

Herbs and Supplements for Sexual Health

There is plenty you can do with herbs and supplements to spark your sex life. Sometimes a lack of libido can be caused by a simple nutritional deficiency or, as I mentioned earlier, chronic dehydration. Something as simple as a vitamin E or zinc deficiency can contribute to low sex drive. In fact, having too much sex can deplete a man of zinc, which will in turn reduce sex drive. This seems to be nature's built-in mechanism for moderation.

Of course my first recommendation for a healthy sex life is to follow the dietary and lifestyle changes in the previous chapter, "Prescription for a Long and Active Sex Life." But if you need a little extra jump start, something in the vitamin, mineral, amino acid or herb department might be just the ticket. (Foods, supplements and herbs for prostate health will be covered in detail in the next section of the book.)

SUPPLEMENTS FOR SEXUAL HEALTH

As I mentioned briefly in the last chapter, stress will lower sex drive in even a very physically healthy man. Constantly releasing stress hormones from the adrenal glands will deplete sex hormones. Both stress hormones and sex hormones, called steroid hormones, are made from cholesterol and use the same biochemical pathways. If adrenal hormones become exhausted, the sex hormones aren't far behind. Stress also interferes with digestion, making your body less able to absorb and utilize the nutrients you are getting from food and vitamins. And meanwhile, the stress hormones raise LDL cholesterol levels, adding insult to injury. You can support your adrenal glands by reducing stress, exercising, getting plenty of sleep, eating properly and taking some vitamins.

There are many steps along the pathway to manufacturing your steroid hormones, and each one requires very specific vitamin and mineral co-factors. Some of the most important co-factor vitamins and minerals include the B vitamins, vitamin E, vitamin C, magnesium and zinc. Also necessary, although in smaller amounts, are iron, molybdenum and manganese. One researcher gave 35 infertile men 1,000 mg of vitamin C daily. Just the addition of this vitamin significantly increased their sperm counts. Vitamin E is the antioxidant of choice in the reproductive organs, protecting them from oxidation reactions.

Zinc

A man's semen contains very high concentrations of zinc. It is estimated that when a young man ejaculates, he loses 1.4 mg of zinc. Low levels of zinc are correlated with infertility and low sex drive. The mineral selenium works with zinc in the male reproductive system, and low selenium is correlated with a low sperm count. Americans are chronically deficient in selenium because of our mineral-depleted soil, so this is an important mineral to be taking every day as a vitamin. Selenium is found naturally in deep green vegetables, onions, tomatoes and whole grains.

Lecithin

Another nutrient found in high concentrations in semen is lecithin, an essential fatty substance found in the membranes of every cell in the body. Lecithin protects cells from oxidation, keeps them flexible and helps dissolve cholesterol in the blood. It is a primary component of brain cells, nerve cells and muscle cells. High concentrations of lecithin are found in the testicles. Lecithin is made of the B vitamins choline and inositol, and linoleic acid, an essential fatty acid which is found in olive, canola and soy oils. Lecithin is found in meat, egg yolks, whole grains, seeds and soy. You can buy lecithin as granules or in capsules at your health food store. The granules can be eaten plain or sprinkled on cereals, salads and in casseroles (after cooking). It is important to avoid buying rancid lecithin, which will do you more harm than good. It should have a pleasant, nutty smell. I recommend 1 or 2 tablespoons of lecithin daily.

Magnesium

This mineral plays many diverse and important roles in the body, from acting as a co-factor for hundreds of biochemical actions to regulating fluid balance within the cells. Magnesium is important in the production of steroid hormones, including testosterone. Americans tend to be chronically deficient in magnesium, like many other minerals, thanks to processed foods and depleted soils. I recommend that, unless you're eating plenty of fresh, organic vegetables every day, you take 300 mg of magnesium daily. It's best taken in a buffered form, with food, or it can cause diarrhea.

Vitamin A

Vitamin A is so important to a healthy male reproductive system that a deficiency of it is actually known to cause shrinkage of the male sex organs. Vitamin A is essential in maintaining healthy tissues and acts as an antioxidant. Furthermore, you have learned how important the B vitamins are to male health, and most of our B vitamins are derived from protein. Without vitamin A, your body is unable to properly utilize protein. Because vitamin A as a supplement can accumulate in the body and become toxic, most people get their supply by taking beta-carotene, a precursor to the vitamin. You should be getting 15,000 International Units of beta-carotene daily, which is about equal to one carrot. Most yellow and orange vegetables contain plenty of beta-carotene. Vitamin A is found in most fruits and vegetables, fish liver oil and animal liver.

Coenzyme Q10

Coenzyme Q10 (CoQ10) is an enzyme found in the body that can significantly raise your energy levels as well as protect and strengthen the heart, lower blood pressure, and strengthen the immune system. CoQ10 is vital to the production of energy in our cells. Its chemical name is "ubiquinone"—it is ubiquitous, or everywhere, where there is life. Its levels in the human body are highest in the heart and liver. When we are ill or stressed, and as we age, our bodies are less able to produce CoQ10. Many older people whose heart function has degenerated and who try CoQ10, report an almost immediate boost in their energy levels.

CoQ10 should come as a powder in a capsule, and be a deep yellow color. The purity and quality of CoQ10 does vary, and since it's not a cheap supplement, it pays to get a high quality brand. I recommend

30 to 90 mg a day to boost energy and strengthen the heart.

HERBS FOR SEXUAL HEALTH

There are three major categories of herbs for male sexual health. The first category is herbs that tone, strengthen and rejuvenate the male reproductive system, and bring an overall sense of energy. In Chinese medicine these are called "yang" herbs. Yang is a way of describing male energy. These herbs could be thought of as tonic herbs.

The second category of herbs are those that directly stimulate sexual energy and erections, which I'll call stimulatory herbs.

The third category of herbs are those that improve blood flow and circulation in general.

TONIC HERBS

Ashwagandha

Ashwagandha is an herb used in Ayurvedic medicine, often called Indian ginseng. As well as being an immune system booster, improving memory and learning ability, it is used specifically to treat male impotence and infertility. In Ayurvedic medicine it is taken as a root powder in warm milk.

Astralagus

Astralagus is widely used in China as a tonic herb that brings up the energy and increases metabolism. It strengthens the body, increases appetite, builds immune function, improves endurance, improves digestion, and supports such important organs as the adrenals, kidneys and liver. In studies astralagus was shown to improve sperm motility in a test tube. It can be taken as a tincture, a tea, or in capsules, 500 to 1500 mg daily.

Ginseng

Ginseng root is another plant medicine widely used all over Asia, especially in China and Korea. It has been extensively studied, and its properties are so unique that a new term was coined to describe it: "adaptogen," meaning an herb that balances whatever is out of balance in the body. If blood pressure is low, ginseng will raise it; if high, ginseng will lower it. Ginseng is a very stimulating herb, but without the "buzz" associated with caffeine and ephedrine, which also have the effect of constricting blood vessels. Ginseng helps stabilize blood sugar, lowers cholesterol, improves liver function, and is used extensively in China to support people who have been weakened by illness. Some studies show that ginseng increases sperm production and the production of testosterone, and promotes the growth of the testes.

There are many types of ginseng, but the one most studied and widely available is *Panax ginseng*, originally from China. Siberian ginseng has similar properties. The major active ingredient in ginseng is a group of steroid-like substances called ginsenosides. The amount of ginsenosides in various ginseng preparations varies considerably. Look for a standardized product or one that guarantees its ginsenoside content.

STIMULATORY HERBS

Yohimbe

Yohimbe is the only herb known to have a directly aphrodisiac effect, but it should be used with caution.

The yohimbe tree is the source of an extract called yohimbine, the only herbal substance available by a doctor's prescription for treating impotence. However, this does not mean it is safe or effective for everyone. Yohimbe can raise blood pressure, can interact with many types of drugs, including antihistamines, alcohol, tranquilizers and sedatives. Some herbalists believe it can aggravate an inflamed prostate gland. If you decide to try yohimbe, I suggest you do it under the supervision of a health-care professional, and be very cautious. It could be good for what ails you, or it could do you more harm than good. If you purchase it at a health food store, buy a reputable brand, because its quality can vary widely. Follow the directions on the bottle.

Damiana

The leaves of the damiana plant have a long history of use as an aphrodisiac in Central America. It is thought to strengthen the nervous system, support the manufacture of hormones, and acts as an antidepressant. Some researchers believe damiana irritates the urethra slightly, thus sensitizing the penis and making it more responsive to stimulation. Its aphrodisiac action may also have to do with stimulating the production of testosterone, or mimicking the action of testosterone. In Mexico damiana is sold as a liqueur called Creme de Damiana. A tea made from damiana is a common drink in Central America.

HERBS THAT IMPROVE CIRCULATION AND BLOOD FLOW

Ginkgo Biloba

Ginkgo biloba is an ancient Chinese herb that comes from one of the most ancient species of trees on the planet. The Chinese have been using ginkgo leaf medicinally for at least 5,000 years. They prize ginkgo leaves for their ability to improve blood flow to the brain, open up congested lungs, and improve blood flow to the extremities.

In the past decade or so, ginkgo has been the subject of over 300 scientific studies. It is one of the best-selling medicines in Europe, sold to an estimated 10 million people there every year. GBE, a standardized ginkgo biloba extract, is a government-approved medicine in Germany and is covered by health insurance there. In general, ginkgo's healing abilities have to do with improving circulation and increasing the flow of oxygen to the brain and extremities.

In addition to promoting circulation to the extremities, ginkgo improves microcirculation, which is the blood flow into the tiny capillaries. Ginkgo relieves the symptoms of peripheral vascular disease, such as pains in the legs at night, cramps, numbness and impotence.

The effects of ginkgo do not generally show up after a single dose. It is not used in massive quantities but in repeated doses that can produce beneficial effects over a relatively long period of time. The best way to take ginkgo is in a standardized liquid extract. GBE is a concentrated and semi-purified extract designed to enhance ginkgo's health benefits and provide a consistent level of ginkgolides, the most active principles.

I recommend that you find a GBE extract with at least 24 percent ginkgo flavoglycosides. You can take 2-3 tablets daily with food, or use the liquid preparations in a dosage of 1-3 droppersful up to 3 or 4 times a day, but check the label for recommendations.

Cayenne

Cayenne is one of those versatile herbs that serves as a wonderful spice, a good source of nutrition, and as a powerful healing agent. Capsicum peppers and chili peppers have similar properties. The ingredient in peppers that makes them hot, called capsaicin, is widely used in alternative medicine and in Asian medicine.

Chili peppers are also high in vitamin A, the carotenoids such as beta-carotene, calcium, phosphorus, iron, potassium, thiamine, riboflavin and niacin. It is helpful for male sexual health because it effectively stimulates circulation.

As a bonus, regular use of cayenne can reduce levels of "bad" LDL cholesterol and relieve the pain of arthritis. Studies have shown that capsaicin also reduces triglyceride levels, lowers blood pressure and raises metabolism, making it easier to burn fat and lose weight.

You can add cayenne to your food, or take it in capsule form.

PART II:
Keeping Your Prostate Healthy Naturally

CHAPTER 5

Is Your Prostate Healthy?

After leading a prostate-healthy lifestyle, the next most important part of good prostate health is knowing when you're having prostate troubles. There are three basic types of prostate disease: benign prostatic hypertrophy or enlargement (BPH), prostatitis, and cancer of the prostate. You can self-diagnose up to a point, but only a thorough medical examination can precisely determine the condition of the prostate. However, when you go to a mainstream doctor for a medical exam of your prostate, you should be thoroughly versed on the subject, or you may wind up getting more treatment than you need. Your best bet is to find a naturopath, an M.D. with a focus on natural health, an osteopath or a chiropractor.

Mainstream doctors in the United States are only just beginning to accept findings that show the role of nutrition, lifestyle and environment in prostate gland health. Therefore it is in your interests to find a doctor you trust who does keep up with the latest data. A good doctor will agree that prostate trouble is not an inevitable part of growing old, and that a conservative approach is the best approach nearly all the time.

A BRIEF REVIEW OF PROSTATE ANATOMY

The prostate is a gland in men located at the neck of the bladder and urethra (the tube through which urine and semen pass on the way out of the body).

When a male is born, the prostate is about the size of a grain of rice, and by the time he's in his twenties it's about the size and shape of a chestnut. Starting at puberty, the gland produces a milky fluid that mixes with semen during ejaculation. The fluid is designed to prevent infection in the urethra, increase sperm motility (movement) and increase the alkalinity of the vagina.

The prostate stays about the same size until the age when some male hormones begin to decline (in most men, their fifties), and the prostate begins to grow again. This is called benign prostatic hypertrophy (BPH). If the gland grows too much, it can begin to create problems.

IS YOUR PROSTATE HEALTHY? TAKE THE TEST

You used to be in line at the urinal wondering how that guy at the trough could take so long . . . now you're the one. You're holding up the line while your prostate is holding up the flow. The prostate is well positioned to pile on this kind of pressure. Nestling at the base of the bladder, the prostate encircles the urethra, the tube leading from the bladder. Prostate gland enlargement squeezes the urethra, blocking the flow of urine and creating a list of possible symptoms.

Signs of Possible Prostate Trouble

√ Coaxing, waiting—it takes a while to get the stream started.

√ Weak flow, some stopping and starting—the stream is not very strong, drying and starting up again on its own, a condition known as *intermittency.*

√ Dribbling—at the end of urination, a little involuntary flow continues.

√ Frequency—the need to urinate often, even shortly after urinating, especially at night when it is known as *nocturia*.

√ Lack of relief—often the bladder feels unemptied as urination fails to bring complete relief.

√ Urgency—the need to urinate is strong, particularly at night.

√ Swollen bladder—often noticeable when it causes abdominal swelling.

√ Burning sensation—on urination—this can be a sign of infection, often stemming from prostate-caused bladder restriction.

Half of all men in the U.S. over the age of 40 will experience prostate enlargement. In some men it goes virtually unnoticed, and in others it causes some or all of the above-listed problems.

HOW THE PROSTATE GLAND CAUSES URINATION PROBLEMS

Problems with urination can occur even without any prostate involvement. Inhibition about urinating in public, kidney trouble and simple bladder infections can all cause difficulty. There is a very good chance that the prostate gland is a factor in persistent problems, however, once middle age is reached.

The overgrowth of prostate tissues means that the gland begins to push against the structures nearest to it. The inner prostate tissues begin to choke the neck of the urethra, restricting the flow of urine from the bladder. This eventually results in difficulty starting the flow of urine. It can also bring about a stop/start, weak flow of urine.

Growth of the outer or inner tissue of the prostate often leads to overall enlargement, causing the gland to begin to push against the bladder itself. This pressure can trigger the urge to urinate. Pressure leads to blockage of the bladder. The bladder fails to empty completely, urination feels unsatisfactory and the need to urinate becomes frequent. The conditions are compounded since the inner prostate is restricting urine flow, also making it difficult to empty the bladder.

When urine is trapped in the bladder it becomes a breeding ground for bacteria, and infection can result. Infection produces a burning sensation on urination, and bladder pain. Aside from infection, the bladder can swell, often seen as abdominal swelling. Blockage of the bladder can also lead to stiffening of its muscular wall as it compensates for the pressure exerted by the prostate gland. If the bladder wall becomes less flexible, the volume of urine exerts a greater pressure than usual, creating another prostate gland-related reason why the urge to urinate is felt more often, particularly at night.

Some men resort to diuretic drugs in an attempt to resolve urinary problems caused by prostate enlargement. This is a bad idea, since the trouble is essentially a blockage which cannot be flushed away. In fact, diuretics will usually only aggravate conditions, as the poor bladder is put under even greater pressure with no relief possible. That said, there are specific diuretic herbal remedies which also have other healing properties that can be of help in the case of an inflamed prostate. For straightforward urinary trouble, stick to healthy food and selected supplements.

The average man can go four to five hours between trips to the bathroom, for a total of five to six trips in 24 hours. Men who drink diuretics such as coffee, or simply take in a lot of fluids, urinate more frequently.

Cold weather causes increased frequency as blood vessels constrict and less blood circulates, creating less demand for water, which is therefore excreted. Cold also makes bladder muscles constrict, which increases the pressure of its contents, producing the urge to urinate at smaller volumes than usual.

Age can bring increased frequency as the kidneys require more water to flush out excess salt. Old age can also bring a slower flow rate if musculature becomes "baggy" or weakened.

OTHER SYMPTOMS OF PROSTATE PROBLEMS

Aside from urinary problems, enlargement of the prostate gland is usually pain-free. However, there are a few other symptoms that can indicate prostate problems, that every man should be aware of.

If the prostate itself becomes inflamed, it can cause a dull, constant ache between the anus and the back of the scrotum. Pain can also radiate to the groin, the back and legs.

Prostate blockage can cause infection in the urinary tract. The infection can be carried to a kidney, which will cause pain in one side of the back below the lower kidneys. Pain from a kidney infection can also be felt in the testicle on the same side. Painful testicle infection itself can occur when infection travels from the prostate gland.

Prostate or bladder infection can cause pain in the lower abdomen. Most lower abdominal pain associated with the prostate gland occurs with retention of urine. The bladder becomes overfull and painfully distended over the course of a few days.

Blood at the beginning or end of the urinary stream is often due to problems with the prostate or urethra. Conditions arising with the kidneys or bladder tend to cause blood in the entire urinary stream. Blood is also sometimes seen in semen and usually stems from infection of the seminal vesicles or of the prostate. Always seek medical advice for these sorts of symptoms as soon as possible. A good doctor will investigate possible prostatic origins as an underlying cause.

CHAPTER 6

Benign Prostate Enlargement (or BPH)

Thomas Jefferson and Benjamin Franklin were both reportedly afflicted with prostate enlargement. No matter who you are, if you're a man and you live long enough, your aging prostate gland will grow. Commonly called prostate enlargement, this condition is the most common one afflicting the prostate gland. The technical term is "benign prostatic hyperplasia" or "hypertrophy," meaning abnormal, nonmalignant overgrowth of the prostate gland. The term is abbreviated to BPH.

BPH means what it says—the condition is benign, or not harmful. It is not cancer. If the condition does not cause other problems, it might even pass unnoticed. BPH can cause urinary problems and it can be a precursor of prostate inflammation and prostate cancer, so it's worth paying attention to and treating if you begin to have symptoms.

In BPH, glandular cells in the inner portion of the prostate, called the transition zone, begin to live longer than usual and develop lumpy nodules. At the same time, the muscular tissue surrounding the gland begins to tighten. Because the prostate gland surrounds the urethra, the tube from the bladder, the nodules can obstruct the flow of urine. The urethra is further squeezed by the tightened prostate muscle. About 20 percent of men with BPH do not experience urinary trouble because the inner nodules are lateral; that is, they grow sideways into the gland. This "silent" development of BPH may continue until the exterior of the prostate has enlarged to the point where it obstructs the bladder itself. Another 50 percent of men with BPH suffer with middle lobe enlargement, the term for the growth of tissue outward, exerting pressure all around the urethra. Middle and lateral lobe growth is seen in 30 percent of men with BPH. These differences in the way the prostate gland enlarges are the reason why the actual size of the gland is often unrelated to the seriousness of symptoms.

THE CAUSES OF BPH

The biochemical processes that result in BPH are quite involved and the subject of considerable research. Most researchers speculate that, with age, testosterone levels fall, levels of other hormones, including estrogen, increase slightly and the aging prostate gland becomes more hormone-sensitive. Increased hormone sensitivity results in chemical messages to cells to live longer. Other chemicals, called growth factors, produced by prostate cells begin to send messages which encourage glandular cells to grow, form lumpy tissue and secrete less, while the signal to muscle tissue is to tighten.

In addition, prolactin, a hormone secreted by the pituitary gland in the brain, increases the uptake of testosterone. Prolactin also stimulates the action of the enzyme which converts testosterone to a more powerful form. The converted testosterone then triggers unwanted messages to prostate cells. Prolactin levels increase with beer consumption and stress, which is why it is advisable to reduce both to prevent or reduce BPH.

BPH is seldom seen in men below the age of 40 or in men who lose their testes, which produce testosterone, before puberty. Studies at Johns Hopkins University show there is also probably a genetic factor at play in about seven percent of BPH cases. The research looked at men aged 64 and younger with notable prostate enlargement. It was found that relatives of men with early onset of BPH were four times more likely to need prostate surgery. For brothers, the rate was six times.

A major five-year Harvard Medical School study of 25,000 men revealed that a large waistline goes along with a 75 percent increase in urinary symptoms after the age of 50. Adding seven inches round the waist was enough to cause problems. The researchers believe excess abdominal fat can press against the prostate gland, which in turn chokes off urine flow. The scientists also suggest that, since getting fat raises estrogen levels and lowers testosterone levels, it could also influence BPH itself.

A growing body of evidence shows that BPH is affected by nutrition. Studies show a healthy, high-fiber diet and specific supplements can hold off or relieve BPH. If you apply proven natural approaches to BPH, you may well avoid the possibility of considerable trauma from surgery and the side effects of drugs used to treat prostate enlargement.

BPH IS A 20TH-CENTURY PROBLEM

Since the beginning of the 20th century, men in their mid to late forties have been running a 20 percent risk of BPH. One in two men aged 60 or over suffers prostate enlargement, and an estimated 80 percent aged 80 and over have developed the condition. Over $3 billion a year is spent on hospital care and surgery for prostate problems in the United States.

For many men, though, BPH is highly preventable and treatable without surgery or hospitalization. Research and clinical trials continue to prove the effectiveness of nutritional treatment and simple therapies. Surgery is not the inevitable fate of someone with BPH. What's more, your risk of developing problematic BPH doesn't have to be the luck of the draw. Good diet, exercise and sensible use of supplements will all help you buck recent statistical trends.

It's important to keep in mind that simple enlargement of the prostate gland does not need treatment. Treatment for BPH is recommended by doctors only when it causes serious related problems. Surgery to remove excess tissue has so far been the most common course taken when symptoms are serious or related conditions develop. The technical term for any procedure which cuts away prostate gland tissue is "prostatectomy," which takes the form of several types of surgical operation. The average age of men who have a prostatectomy is 70, showing again that prostate trouble is a disease associated with longevity.

As most prostate patients are elderly, they frequently suffer from other conditions which limit the types of treatment that may be applicable. Sometimes physicians will advise the uses of catheters or stents to relieve bladder problems caused by BPH rather than operate on the prostate itself.

For the vast majority of men, symptoms are mild enough that even if BPH is diagnosed, the course advised is just watchful waiting. Your physician may advise limited fluid intake before bed and steer you away from certain drugs such as decongestants which can worsen BPH. But there is more you can do, which I'll tell you about in detail.

Here are some very inspiring reasons to prevent prostate problems:

Possible Side Effects of Prostate Surgery

- "Dry" ejaculation (which does not affect the pleasure of an orgasm) occurs in about 75 to 90 percent of patients.
- Failure of symptoms to improve is seen in about ten percent of cases.
- Infections occur in about ten percent of men.
- About five to ten percent of men have a loss of erection or impotence.
- Transfusions are needed in about five percent of cases.
- Urethral scarring happens in about five percent of patients.
- Serious or permanent incontinence occurs in one percent of patients.

DRUGS FOR BPH

Drugs developed for prostate enlargement are not very effective and tend to have unpleasant side effects. BPH drugs work in two ways: they either interfere with the hormones that trigger prostate cell growth, or they relax prostate muscle tissue to relieve its pressure on the urethra. Neither of these approaches tackles the underlying causes of the hormonal action seen in BPH, which is why they do not cure the condition.

HERBAL REMEDIES FOR BPH

Thanks to the wisdom and practices of native peoples in countries like Africa and America, several effective herbal treatments exist for BPH. These plant-based remedies have been shown in studies to be more effective, safer and cheaper than modern BPH drugs. Your pocketbook and your prostate will benefit when you

use these simple, yet powerful extracts. Backed up by
sensible diet and supplements, herbs are a valuable
part of a comprehensive BPH treatment plan.

Herbs make powerful medicine. If you are taking
any medication or have been diagnosed with cancer,
heart problems of any kind, hypertension, impotence
due to nerve damage, or any other major condition,
always check any form of self-treatment you are considering with your physician.

Saw Palmetto (Serenoa repens)

According to folk history, the small, wrinkly, reddish-
brown to black berries of the saw palmetto tree make
a good aphrodisiac. In fact, it is an overall tonic for
the male reproductive system, and formed part of the
diet of some native Americans. Early herbalists used
saw palmetto berries to increase testicle function and
to treat prostate conditions. The tree itself is a palm
tree, but grows only six to ten feet tall. It is native to
the dunes and coasts of Florida, Texas and Georgia.

Several clinical studies published in the 1980s in
professional journals demonstrate the value of saw palmetto extract in treating almost 90 percent of BPH
patients studied. One trial compared men with BPH
taking saw palmetto extract with others taking a placebo. After just 28 days, of the 110 men studied, those
using the extract saw a 40 to 50 percent improvement
in symptoms. Those on a placebo showed no significant improvement. The results were supported in rat-
ings by both patients and doctors.

A three-month study of 350 men taking 160 mg of
saw palmetto extract twice daily showed an 88 percent
improvement in symptoms within 90 days. This favorable
result was echoed in the objective findings. Remark-
able improvements were obtained in all measurements, including urinary flow, flow rate and prostate

size. Another important finding was the self-rating for quality of life. The number of men who considered themselves unhappy dropped from 18.5 percent to 2.4 percent, while those who felt satisfied with life numbered only 9.7 percent at the beginning of the trial, but jumped to 36.8 percent by the end. As well as demonstrating the value of saw palmetto extract, these findings show just how much BPH symptoms can badly affect mental outlook. Relieving the condition can make a big change for the better in a man's life.

Saw Palmetto or Modern Drugs?

The good results with saw palmetto for almost all patients in clinical trials are also encouraging because they were achieved without any side effects or toxicity. Safe use goes for both the extract and for eating the berries themselves. This is in contrast to Proscar (finasteride), a prescription drug approved by the FDA for use in 1992 to treat BPH. A year's course of Proscar has been shown to work in less than 50 percent of patients. When trial results are compared, patients using saw palmetto extract show greater improvement in symptoms at three months than men using Proscar. Furthermore, Proscar caused impotence in 3.7 percent of men and decreased libido in 3.3 percent. Pregnant women are advised not to handle the drug or expose themselves to the semen of men who are taking it. Proscar is also four times more expensive than saw palmetto. It's clear that natural saw palmetto is a much safer and effective remedy for BPH than this expensive drug of the '90s.

How Saw Palmetto Relieves BPH

The compounds in saw palmetto extract are known as antagonists to the effects of the form of testosterone which initiates BPH. They work in two ways: by inhibiting the formation of the converted testosterone (dihydrotestosterone or DHT) and help block it from binding to receptor sites on cells. By inhibiting the binding of DHT, saw palmetto also encourages its breakdown and excretion—good news for the aging prostate. Herbalists have also found that saw palmetto has a mild sedative effect, which is helpful to patients getting over nighttime urination problems.

If you take saw palmetto in a tincture form, be prepared for the strong taste, which is disagreeable to many. At least 10 to 20 grams of the raw fruit would have to be eaten twice a day to take in enough of the active chemicals. You can also take it in capsule form.

Pygeum Africanum

An evergreen, pygeum grows to more than 100 feet tall in Madagascar and on the high plateaus of central and southern Africa, where it is native. The tribes of Natal create infusions of the dark brown or gray pygeum bark to treat bladder pains and urinary difficulty, familiar symptoms to men with BPH. Other countries have been slow to catch on. The herb was only introduced to Europe in the 1960s after researchers observed its effectiveness among native peoples. It wasn't long, however, before European journals began to publish exciting studies verifying pygeum as a valuable BPH treatment. European men have benefited, as now 81 percent of all doctors' prescriptions for BPH in France are for extract of *Pygeum africanum*, where it relieves symptoms for more than half of all BPH patients.

Yet in America, doctors are only just beginning to learn about pygeum, where it has been viewed only as a "health food."

Why Pygeum is used for BPH

Like saw palmetto berries, the bark of pygeum contains fatty acids and sterols. These act to inhibit the formation of the prostate growth stimulant DHT. They also help to balance prostate testosterone levels, and the sterols help to reduce prostate inflammation. The compounds in pygeum act in a slightly different way from those in saw palmetto. They are not quite as good at reducing symptoms, and some men do not tolerate them as well, experiencing nausea or stomach pains. There is not as much information about objective measurements of symptoms with use of pygeum as there is for saw palmetto. However, the biochemical actions of pygeum appear to be complementary as well as overlapping to those of saw palmetto and the two herbs are often taken together. This is advisable, since pygeum also improves the quality and quantity of prostate secretions which is something saw palmetto does not accomplish.

Analysis of the studies of outpatients since the mid-'70s shows that pygeum lessens symptoms and clinical signs of BPH, particularly in cases detected early on in their development. Look for extracts standardized to 14 percent sterols.

Flower Pollen Extract

In Europe, flower pollen extract has been used to treat BPH and prostate inflammation for over 25 years. The main product used is called Cernilton, produced in Sweden and available in health food stores in the U.S. Published clinical studies show Cernilton is probably most effective in the treatment of prostate inflammation, but can also be helpful in treating BPH. A report in the *Swedish Medical Journal* described a small one-year trial using Cernilton that resulted in the prostate returning to normal size in five out of ten patients. The most improvement was seen in patients with inflamed prostates. None of the studies found any side effects.

Pollen is a rich supply of vitamins and minerals, trace elements and carbohydrates. It also contains fatty acids, flavonoids and protein. The mechanisms are unclear, but the effects of these agents are to reduce inflammation, contract the bladder and relax the urethra. The result is less pain and eased urinary symptoms. Use pollen with care, as some people are allergic to different types.

Panax Ginseng

Ginseng is an ancient oriental herb, used for centuries as a male tonic. A study of male rats showed that ginseng increased testosterone while decreasing prostate gland weight. One of the effects of lowered testosterone levels seen in the aging male body is a decreased uptake of zinc. Increasing testosterone would in theory lead to higher levels of zinc, which is proven to be effective in reducing the size of enlarged prostates.

If you decide to use ginseng, be careful to select a genuine *Panax ginseng* product standardized for its "ginsenoside" content, as ginseng quality is highly variable.

HOW TO USE HERBAL REMEDIES FOR BPH

Using herbs to treat BPH, you'll generally begin to notice an effect within a few days or weeks, but for some men they can take up to three months to take effect. The following guidelines should help:

- **Saw Palmetto.** Take 160 mg of liposterolic (85-95 percent) extract twice daily (equivalent to about 10 gms of raw berries twice daily). If no result occurs from using saw palmetto alone for three months, pygeum can be used instead, or you can try taking them together.

- **Pygeum Africanum.** Take 50 to 100 mg of extract twice daily (almost always available as a pill). The most potent form is a 70:1 extract, but many men see good results with just an 8:1 extract. Studies show saw palmetto has a slightly stronger effect on symptoms, but pygeum also improves prostate secretions. For this reason the two can be used in combination.

- **Flower Pollen Extract.** Take two tablets of Cernilton or similar products three times daily. Avoid if allergic to pollen.

- **Panax Ginseng.** Take the dried root, 2-4 grams three times daily, or extracts equivalent to 25 to 50 mg ginsenosides daily.

CHAPTER 7

Prostate Inflammation

There are other prostate problems that don't fit under the BPH category, and which can usually be treated successfully with noninvasive, natural methods.

First, do not be confused by the term "prostatosis." This is medico-speak for "a condition of the prostate," often used when a doctor does not know what is wrong.

PROSTATITIS

Prostatitis means inflammation of the prostate gland. It is a common ailment of young men prone to urinary tract infections, while older men are prone to prostate enlargement. The usual symptoms of an inflamed prostate include discomfort in and around the gland, usually accompanied by acute urinary symptoms such as burning and increased and urgent need to urinate. Pain from an inflamed prostate gland can be transmitted around the anus and scrotum, the groin, the lower back, lower abdomen and the legs. Prostatitis can also cause pain on ejaculation.

Zinc dissolved in prostate fluid exhibits antibacterial action, and levels have been found to be as low as one-tenth of normal in men with prostatitis. It's not surprising, then, that studies show that prostatitis symptoms can resolve with zinc supplementation. Zinc should be taken in a readily absorbable form such as zinc picolinate, and not for too long at high doses.

To prevent and relieve prostatitis, consumption of foods rich in zinc such as herring and pumpkin seeds is a good idea.

A mainstream treatment of prostatitis can be problematic, because even a normal prostate gland is poorly supplied with blood, making it a tough site for the immune system to defend and for antibiotics to reach. For this reason, recurrences of this type of infection are common. Some mainstream urologists have resorted to prescribing a long, six-week term of antibiotic treatment. Such a long course of antibiotics is hard on the body and ignores probable contributory nutritional deficiencies that leave the immune system underpowered. A better path may be a more standard two-week course of antibiotics backed up by supplements, including vitamins C and E and zinc. Also ensure that your diet is high in fiber and nutrients. Cut out coffee and other prostate irritants, and drink plenty of clean water. Vitamin B-complex and probiotic supplements like acidophilus are also a must with antibiotics.

Nonbacterial prostatitis, the term for prostate inflammation not caused by bacteria, is the most common type of prostatitis, but it has doctors puzzled. Patients suffer the same symptoms as chronic bacterial prostatitis, but their urine shows no sign of infection and antibiotics have no effect. In addition, most sufferers have never had a urinary tract infection. The pain involved and white blood cells in the prostatic fluid are the main signs of prostatitis.

Herbs to Treat Prostate Infection and Inflammation

- **Bearberry.** Traditionally used as a diuretic, but as it contains flavonoids and a substance called arbutin which converts in the human body to hydroquinone, it is also a urinary disinfectant. Hydroquinone is poisonous at high doses, but bearberry is safe for short-term treatment of prostate gland infection.

- **Couch grass.** Also known as witch grass, among other names, this herb is used specifically to treat prostatitis as well as urinary tract infections and urinary stones. Couch grass is rich in oils, and contains vitamins A and B, and other valuable compounds such as iron. It is a soothing diuretic with antibiotic properties.
- **Echinacea.** Known for its immune-boosting properties, which are due to its mix of essential oils and other potent plant chemicals. Echinacea is used in the treatment of infections generally.
- **Goldenseal.** Is effective in treating urinary and kidney infections and stones. Goldenseal has cleansing actions that stem from its mixture of essential oils, flavonoids, tannins and saponins.
- **Horsetail.** Offers a storehouse of minerals useful in treating prostatitis, BPH, cystitis and urinary stones. Saponins are also found in this herb, probably contributing their antimicrobe and hormone-mimicking properties when horsetail is used as remedy.

CHAPTER 8

Prostate Cancer

Fear and confusion surround the topic of prostate cancer for many men. However, the statistics and research provide a great deal of reassurance. Even though more than half of all men experience prostate enlargement, only 13 percent of men develop threatening cancer of the prostate gland and only 2 to 3 percent will die of the condition. Prostate cancer is age-related, developing almost exclusively in men over 50 years of age. More than 80 percent of men diagnosed with prostate cancer are over the age of 65.

An analysis of population studies and experimental evidence shows that several dietary factors increase the risk of developing prostate cancer. A high intake of refined sugar, animal protein and animal fat, and a lack of carotenes, also known as carotenoids (found in carrots and other orange and yellow vegetables), were the most significant. Clearly then, a diet rich in fruit and vegetables, and low in meat and animal fats, should offer some protection against prostate cancer.

Heredity can confer up to a 50 percent risk of developing prostate cancer. This risk is seen in men when prostate cancer has occurred in three generations of their family, or in men with three or more close relatives, father or brother, who suffer from the disease. This accounts for only about five percent of prostate cancers.

Prostate cancer is the most common form of cancer in men, but it lies behind lung cancer as their main cause of cancer deaths. Only two to three percent of men die of prostate cancer. Compare that to the 47 percent of American men who die of heart disease. Any man can lessen his risk of prostate cancer by adopting a healthy lifestyle. Diet is almost certainly a major reason why there is less incidence of prostate cancer in countries like Japan, particularly since rates of this condition increase in Japanese men whose diet becomes more westernized.

THE TWO FORMS OF PROSTATE CANCER

Like all cancers, prostate cancer consists of undifferentiated cells that grow out of control. Normal growth checks have little or no effect on cancer cells, which can invade and destroy normal cells. A study of 100 tissue samples removed in surgery shows that the size of a prostate tumor is related to how dangerous it is. Scientists found that tumors less than 1 cubic centimeter (just under half an inch) rarely spread. Most tumors under 3.5 cubic centimeters remained inside the prostate. The bigger a tumor, however, the more aggressive it becomes. Tumors over 5 cubic centimeters are more difficult to treat.

Early prostate cancer is slow-growing, often taking two to four years or longer to double in size. To reach one cubic centimeter a tumor has to double at least thirty times, and it would be at about this point that a tumor could be felt by a doctor. Due to this growth pattern, prostate cancer is considered to exist in two forms:

"Incidental," "histologic" and "latent" are terms for microscopic cancer seen on slides, usually at autopsy. This form is thought to affect about 60 to 70 percent of all men over 80 years old, going undetected in most. This gives physicians the problem of whether or not to treat incidental cancer when discovered since it could easily continue to exist without causing any problems. In the younger man, early development of a tumor is believed to be a sign that the cancer is likely to evolve into a threatening form. Older men may well die of other causes long before their prostate cancer becomes a problem.

The second type of prostate cancer is called "clinical," "clinically significant," "advanced," and "malignant." These terms refer to cancer which may spread to other parts of the body. The nearby seminal vesicles, bladder, urethra and pelvic side walls are common sites for prostate cancer which has begun to spread. From these sites it can be carried via the lymph system and the bloodstream to sites such as bones or lungs. It can grow "silently" or cause symptoms. Clinical prostate cancer is two and one-half times less common than the incidental kind. There is a genetic connection for clinical prostate cancer. Having a father or brother with the disease means a man's risk of developing it is two times greater than normal and often leads to earlier affliction. Prostate cancer in three generations of either parent's family brings a one-in-two risk of its development.

Another term used in relation to prostate cancer is "localized." This refers to cancer that has not developed beyond the prostate gland. Prostate cancer can remain in the gland indefinitely, which is why many elderly men can have prostate cancer but die of other causes. Removal of the prostate gland is the most extreme treatment for localized prostate cancer, and is termed a "radical prostatectomy." Localized cancer usually takes two or three years to double in size.

The environmental factor is important when considering the two forms of prostate cancer. This is shown in studies of Japanese and American men. Incidental prostate cancer is as common in both groups of men, and both groups have the same lifespan of 74 years.

Yet far fewer men in Japan die of prostate cancer. Rates of prostate cancer death in Japanese men who move to Hawaii or California shoot up to American levels. The major factor here seems to be diet. The effects of diet, nutrients and other agents are thought to act in a way which inhibits the growth of cancer beyond its first stage, called initiation. It is the further stages of cancer, promotion, progression, and metastasis, that are seen less commonly in Japanese men.

SYMPTOMS OF PROSTATE CANCER

Most prostate cancers, about 72 percent, begin in the outer, "peripheral zone" of the gland, and 8 percent start in the "central zone." The remaining 20 percent begin in the "transition zone," which is where prostate enlargement originates. For this reason and because it is slow-growing in its early stage, prostate cancer, unlike BPH, does not at first cause pressure on the urethra and connected urinary problems. Silent development is typical, and the cancer is often quite advanced once it causes symptoms. Such symptoms include signs of BPH, blood in the urine or semen, less ejaculated fluid, less rigid erections or impotence, and severe pain in the back, pelvis, hips or thighs. It's important to remember that all of these problems can have other causes. If you are experiencing prostate problems, get a thorough annual prostate checkup.

DIAGNOSIS OF PROSTATE TROUBLE

Debate is heated on the subject of diagnosis of prostate gland problems, cancer in particular. Doctors disagree about methods of diagnosis, test results, and the significance of physical signs. Some physicians look for BPH earlier than others, some pathologists have seen cancerous cells where others have not. Studies are ongoing to determine the value of different tests and the way they are used. One of the most important prostate diagnostic tests is the DRE, or digital rectal exam.

Yes, it's time for all those rubber-glove jokes. Women in our culture have long been used to pelvic examinations. Men, on the other hand, tend to have relatively little experience of a physician inserting things into their lower regions. No doubt many men wish that "digital exam" referred to a high-tech electronic procedure. In fact, a digital rectal exam uses a surgically-gloved finger to conduct a basic, but usually effective test of prostate health.

The digital rectal examination is a subjective test and is best performed by a doctor experienced and expert in the procedure. The message again on diagnosing prostate trouble is to seek out a good, likeable physician. It is also important to note that as many as 40 percent of prostate cancers begin in a spot which is inaccessible through this procedure. In some cases, disease can be advanced by the time it is detected through a digital exam. Make sure your physician uses this diagnostic tool with a PSA test. The PSA and digital rectal exam were almost equal in their ability to detect cancers in a study of 2,634 men. However, the different tests did not always find the same tumors. If only one had been used, some cancers would have been missed.

Healthy prostate tissue feels much like the flesh between the first finger and thumb when a fist is made. It is firm and smooth without being solid. The length of tissue felt by the doctor should be no more than about one and a half inches long. The physician will check if the prostate tissue feels hard, lumpy, or soft and mushy. He will also be alert for any enlargement of the gland, which can grow to the size of an orange in some cases. Often, however, the inner prostate tissue has enlarged without causing any external expansion of the gland. For this reason, the digital rectal exam is not a surefire way to diagnose BPH.

A physician may also "milk" the prostate gland during a DRE. Pressure on the gland can push a drop or two of prostate fluid into the urethra. Such drops can be collected when passed through the urethra and checked microscopically for signs of bacterial infection.

It is well worth overcoming any embarrassment or distaste for this simple procedure. It is a useful aid in assessing prostate health.

PSA–the Prostate Specific Antigen Test

This test has become highly controversial in recent years. It has a high rate of false positives—up to 75 percent—meaning that up to 75 percent of the time it will show that a man has prostate cancer when he doesn't. It also has a high false negative rate, meaning it fails to indicate the presence of a cancer. It can also indicate the genuine existence of prostate cancer in elderly men who are unlikely to survive to see the cancer become problematic. Doctors and patients then cannot be sure that treatment would ultimately improve health or life expectancy.

An antigen is a substance which stimulates the production of antibodies by the immune system. Often an antigen is something foreign to the body. Prostatic-specific antigen, however, is a protein secreted almost exclusively by cells of the prostate gland. Its role is to break down coagulated semen. Normally, very little PSA leaks into the blood. Elevated PSA levels can be a sign of BPH, infection and prostatitis. High PSA levels are mainly associated with cancer because it often effectively makes prostate cell walls leaky. However, PSA is prostate-specific, not cancer-specific, so the PSA could be high for any number of reasons besides the

presence of cancer. To complicate matters even further, about one-quarter of men who turn out to have
prostate cancer have *low* PSA levels. In men with PSA
levels between four and ten, about a quarter have cancer. About 65 percent of men with PSA levels over 10
turn out to have cancer. PSA readings alone should
not form the basis of prostate cancer diagnosis. In
fact, older men who get PSA tests and then allow
themselves to undergo surgery have a higher death
rate than men who do nothing. Since prostate cancer
is such a slow-growing cancer, watchful waiting has
been recommended by many highly respected physicians. And while you wait watchfully, there's plenty
you can do with nutrition and lifestyle to reduce your
chances of a serious prostate cancer.

A University of Chicago study published in the New
England Journal of Medicine is an example of the evidence regarding treatment of prostate cancer in men
with overall short life expectancy. The study found
that those expected generally to live only ten years or
less at the time their cancer is detected (i.e., men in
their 70s and 80s) are much more likely to die of
a cause other than untreated prostate cancer. Since
prostate surgery can cause incontinence, impotence
and general weakness, it's highly debatable whether it
will do more harm than good in most cases.

Unless it becomes possible to refine PSA testing,
different tests are advisable to see if results are consistent. The combination of PSA with a digital rectal
exam is recommended. Ultrasound and needle biopsy
can also be used. Each of these tests can pick up cancers the other missed. Surgery should only be under-
taken if serious cancer is a near-certainty.

Ask if your doctor is aware of the latest information
about PSA testing. Does he monitor PSA velocity and
calculate PSA density? Has he heard of PSA level age
ranges? Ask and see if the response is positive, open

and well informed. If it's not and he or she seems over-eager to perform surgery, run the other way and find another doctor!

Remember, only 13 percent of men are diagnosed with prostate cancer and only 2 to 3 percent die of it. What's more, 80 percent of men with prostate cancer are over 65 and most of them die from other causes. Less than one percent of prostate cancers have been found in men younger than 50 and only 16 percent in men aged between 50 and 64. The average age of prostate cancer diagnosis is 72. Confusion arises because, although incidental prostate cancer is believed to exist in about two thirds of all men over 80 years old, wherever they live, diagnosis of advanced, clinical cancer occurs, as mentioned, for only 13 percent.

Prostate enlargement or BPH is much more common, affecting half of all men aged 60. If owners took better care of their prostate glands would these statistics improve? The studies of Japanese men as well as those on particular nutrients and herbs indicate they would. Sound nutrition and a healthy lifestyle can only help guard against prostate trouble.

CHAPTER 9

Nutrition and the Prostate

Are you a hunter-gatherer, driving herds of game, fishing and harvesting your way through life? Or do you drive a car, graze the Internet and hunt down bargains? Along with 20th-century changes in the lifestyle and diet of modern man has come a staggering increase in the incidence of prostate trouble. The medical establishment has held that prostate gland trouble is an inevitable consequence of aging, and more than $3 billion is spent annually on prostate-related surgery. Look to Asia, however, and you'll find a much lower incidence of prostate problems. Even in the Far East, though, rates of prostate disease have risen at the same time as the Asian diet has become increasingly westernized.

While doctors debate the causes of BPH, more and more research points to nutritional connections. Numerous studies show that good nutrition plays an important role in the prevention of and relief from prostate disease. It's a wise prostate health maintenance move to make the dietary changes needed and take supplements selected for their proven effects.

AMINO ACIDS RELIEVE PROSTATE SYMPTOMS

Amino acids have been shown in several studies to relieve many of the symptoms of BPH. For instance, an American study of 45 men with BPH showed that 95 percent of those using three amino acids found relief from or reduction in night-time urination, with a high percentage of alleviation of other symptoms also being achieved. The three amino acids found to be effective are alanine, glycine and glutamic acid. However, the mechanisms at work are unclear and many researchers believe amino acid treatment for prostates only reduces symptoms without curing prostate problems.

CAROTENES, CANCER, INFECTION AND THE PROSTATE

Some studies have shown that a low intake of carotenoids, particularly beta-carotene, adds a significant risk for prostate cancer. Carotenoids are red to yellow plant pigments best known for their antioxidant activity and anticancer properties, and their conversion to vitamin A in the body.

Vitamin A helps the prostate overcome and resist infections by keeping its mucous membranes functioning well. It aids the production of cells that grow tiny hairs called cilia, which trap and sweep out germs and other foreign matter. To increase your intake of these helpful substances, eat lots of yellow-orange fruits and vegetables like carrots, apricots, sweet potatoes, yams and squash. Dark green leafy vegetables, such as kale and spinach, are also excellent carotene sources. Taking a beta-carotene supplement is not a substitute for eating plenty of carotenoid-rich fruits and vegetables!

VITAMIN B6 AND BLADDER STONES

Bladder stones are seen more commonly in parts of the world where a vitamin B6 deficiency is found. A lack of this vitamin increases the excretion of oxalate in urine. Oxalate tends to crystallize easily, forming stones. As BPH often leads to the retention of urine, there is an increased likelihood that stones will form. Taking a good vitamin B-complex supplement is wise insurance against this condition. It also indirectly aids the prostate through the involvement of vitamin B6 in the synthesis and management of hormones and as an aid to the absorption of the critical prostate mineral zinc.

VITAMIN C AND THE PROSTATE GLAND

This is one case where flushing a vitamin down the toilet actually does you good—as long as it's passed through you first! Up to 60 percent of vitamin C consumed ends up in urine. Owing to its beneficial effects on the urinary tract, however, this apparent loss is not a waste at all. Authorities in the United States report that vitamin C is effective against inflammation of the urethra. The body requires higher levels of vitamin C at times of any infection, but it is thought its beneficial effects in the urethra are also due in part to the way high doses of vitamin C increase the acidity of urine. Retention of urine is a common result of BPH that can lead to infection of the bladder and urethra. Retained urine begins to decompose, becoming less acidic. This can also lead to the formation of tiny crystalline stones in the urine which cause pain and irritation. Of course, tackling infection in the urinary tract keeps down the risk of the condition spreading to the prostate and causing prostatitis. Vitamin C as a powerful anti-infectant is also definitely recommended for prostatitis itself.

Include zinc on your supplements list, too, since vitamin C works more efficiently with zinc. The two substances create a very good anti-infection double act for the prostate gland and urinary tract.

VITAMIN D AND THE ULTRAVIOLET
PROSTATE CONNECTION

A study published in the journal *Cancer* found that deaths from prostate cancer in white men were more common in northern areas of the United States. Those areas with greatest sunlight saw the least prostate cancer. These findings also correlate with the fact that prostate cancer rates are lowest in Japan and Hong Kong, and highest in the United States, Canada and Scandinavia. The study suggests that ultraviolet radiation may protect against clinical prostate cancer.

There may also be a link to vitamin D, which is mainly synthesized by the body as a result of exposure to sunlight. Vitamin D is known to be able to inhibit the growth of tumors, preventing them from progressing past the incidental stage.

Japan is not only exposed to more ultraviolet light, the Japanese diet is rich in fish with a high vitamin D content. Research into the ultraviolet connection and prostate cancer has only just begun and much more work needs to be completed before anyone can definitely say that a lack of vitamin D increases the risk of prostate cancer. Of course, overexposure to ultraviolet radiation brings a high risk itself of skin cancer. There would be no harm, though, and possibly some insurance against prostate cancer, in taking a daily ten-minute walk without sunscreen, and returning to a grilled fish dinner!

ESSENTIAL FATTY ACIDS PROMOTE
PROSTATE HEALTH

Pumpkin seeds for virility? There is some truth to folklore from Eastern Europe where pumpkin seeds have long been used as a prostate tonic and remedy. It took until the late 1920s, however, for scientists at the

University of Vienna to discover that men in countries like Bulgaria, the Ukraine and Turkey really did have much lower rates of prostate enlargement.

As well as being an excellent source of zinc, pumpkin seeds are rich in essential fatty acids (EFAs). Among other functions, EFAs regulate hormone action and aid in the breakdown of cholesterol, both of which are linked to prostate problems. A study from a nutritional research foundation in Milwaukee has shown that supplementation with EFAs alone for several weeks reduced or completely relieved prostate enlargement symptoms.

FLAVONOIDS PROTECT AGAINST PROSTATE CANCER

When you eat plenty of fresh fruit, you'll increase the concentration of flavonoids in your blood. The berries and citrus fruits have the highest concentration of flavonoids. Flavonoids—including bioflavonoids and isoflavonoids—are found in the pigmentation of plants and act as powerful antioxidants.

A small study published in *The Lancet* compared the levels of isoflavonoids in the blood of Finnish and Japanese men. Levels in the Japanese men were 110 times higher than those in the Finnish men! The researchers observed that lifelong high blood concentrations of isoflavonoids may explain the low incidence of clinical cancer in Japanese men. One notable ingredient of Japanese traditional diet is soy. Eating soy is one of the best ways to ensure a high intake of flavonoids.

SAPONINS AND POSSIBLE PROSTATE CANCER PROTECTION

Saponins are yet another plant ingredient that may be part of the reason for differences in cancer rates between countries with very different diets. Saponins mimic precursors to steroid hormones. Research at the University of Toronto is showing that the rates of prostate and other cancers are lower where people eat foods richest in saponins. Saponins may well be a supplement of the future. In the meantime, it can only pay to eat plenty of saponin-rich vegetables like beans, spinach, tomatoes, potatoes, alfalfa and even oats.

ZINC FIGHTS BPH

Old wives' tales have it that oysters are an aphrodisiac, and the old wives seem to be right most of the time! Oysters are high in zinc, which is essential to the workings of the male reproductive system.

When it comes to the prostate, zinc is a mineral which inhibits the activity of the enzyme which converts testosterone to its more powerful form. The converted testosterone triggers prostate cells to grow abnormally, resulting in an enlarged prostate. Zinc has also been shown to inhibit the activity of prolactin, the hormone which also stimulates the testosterone-converting enzyme as well as increasing the uptake of testosterone itself.

Most American men are deficient in zinc. You may read in some publications that zinc supplementation does not result in higher levels being found in the prostate. In some cases this may be true. BPH is an older man's disease, and increasing age often brings a lessening of pancreatic function, which is necessary for the absorption of zinc. What's more, the lowered testosterone levels seen in the older man lead to less absorption of zinc in the intestine. Adequate levels of vitamin B6 are needed, too, for the uptake of zinc. What is certain is that there have been many studies showing that zinc does indeed reduce the symptoms of BPH. Measurements by digital rectal exam, endoscopy and X-ray have all shown that treatment with zinc reduces the size of prostate enlargement. It's essential, however, to see that zinc is taken in a readily absorbable form, usually zinc picolinate, and to ensure sound nutrition in general.

Zinc also fights infection and boosts the efficiency of vitamin C. Cut down on alcohol to keep levels up. Eat lots of nuts and seeds, especially pumpkin seeds, and be sure this is one substance on your prostate health supplement list!

HOW MUCH OF ANY SUPPLEMENT SHOULD I TAKE?

It does not follow that, because a substance is beneficial, more is better. Taken at high levels for too long, zinc, for example, will depress the immune system. Illness usually produces an increased need for various nutrients. Individual requirements vary, too, so be prepared to monitor your progress and seek advice from a knowledgeable health-care professional.

Supplements are just that! They are not a substitute for a good, healthy diet, but *are* useful support for one that is not ideal, as well as for modern, fast-paced, highly stressed lifestyles and environments. Note, too, that nutritional substances work in balance with each other, becoming most efficient when general background nutrition is sound. Partly in keeping with this principle, and partly for convenience, formulas have been developed that combine supplements which specifically address prostate trouble. The following quantity guidelines are frequently recommended:

Supplements for a Healthy Prostate

√ **Zinc picolinate.** Take 15-30 mg daily (increase to 60 mg for prostatitis until symptoms subside).

√ **Vitamin B6 (pyridoxine).** —Take 50-100 mg daily.
Always take vitamin B complex, too, when you
take a B vitamin supplement. Some B-complex
"stress" formulas include higher amounts of B6
and B5.

√ **Alanine, glycine, glutamic acid.** Take 200 mg daily
of these amino acids. I prefer you take your glutamic acid in the form of glutamine, which the
body will convert to glutamic acid as needed.

√ **Vitamin C.** Take 1,000 mg three times daily. Increase this triple dose to 2,000 mg at the onset of
prostatitis. Vitamin C intake can be increased
until it causes diarrhea (then back the dose off),
as the body's requirement for this vitamin varies
considerably with illness and stress.

FOODS FOR A HEALTHY PROSTATE

One thing for certain is that a lot of red meat, animal
fats, butter, mayonnaise and creamy salad dressings
are not food for a healthy prostate gland. A Harvard
Medical School study showed that these foods were
most closely linked to a risk of advanced, fatal cancer.
Analysis of dietary and blood sample data from 300
cases, including 126 advanced cases of prostate cancer,
was compared with that from a comparable group of
healthy doctors. Analysis showed that eating meat just
once a week, instead of five times, could lower your
risk of advanced cancer by two to three times. However, consuming high amounts of any of the offending
foods raises blood levels of a type of fatty acid called
alpha-linolenic acid or ALA. It was this fatty acid that
seemed to cause the increased risk, probably through
its enzyme-related activity in the prostate.

Evidence that high cholesterol levels are bad for the
prostate comes from the fact that anticholesterol

drugs have been shown to relieve BPH. In addition, a study from the Metropolitan Hospital in New York found that men with BPH had 80 percent more cholesterol in their blood than men without BPH. Harmful substances are produced when cholesterol breaks down. If the body is deficient in nutrients like vitamins C and E and essential fatty acids, then the harmful cholesterol by-products are not cleared out of the body. Some accumulate in the prostate gland, where they promote BPH. This rules out processed and refined foods, including sugar, and saturated fats in large amounts if BPH is to be avoided.

If fatty, mainly animal based and refined foods are out, what's in? It makes sense to look for examples in countries like Bulgaria and Japan where rates of BPH or prostate cancer are low. The following will all help to keep your prostate in good shape—literally!

Soy. A plant source of complete protein and numerous other valuable nutrients such as flavonoids (plant hormones) and essential fatty acids. Try the different varieties from tofu to tempeh and soy flour to soy drinks. There are lots of different recipes.

Cold-water fish. Salmon, cod, sardines and tuna are an excellent source of vitamin D and essential fatty acids, both of benefit to the prostate. Herring is also high in zinc.

Fresh vegetables. From dark green and leafy to yellow and red to white and creamy, all will keep you well supplied with carotenes, flavonoids and saponins, as well as lots of vitamins and fiber. Fiber is particularly helpful in keeping cholesterol levels down, which is important for the prostate gland.

Fresh fruit. The best for the prostate are the red and yellow kinds from tomatoes (yes, they're a fruit, not a vegetable!), and apricots to strawberries and oranges. A good source of vitamin C, many fruits are high in the plant pigments called flavonoids and carotenoids which are nutritional powerhouses.

Nuts and seeds. A daily handful of nuts and seeds is a good source of protective minerals and essential fatty acids. Pumpkin and sunflower seeds especially will also help keep you topped up with zinc which, like essential fatty acids, is involved with hormone regulation important to prostate health. Zinc also fights and resists prostate related infections.

Whole grains. Wheat, oatmeal, brown rice and other complex carbohydrates help keep your cholesterol levels low and fiber up, both significant aids to the prostate. Oatmeal and wheat bran are also both fairly good sources of zinc, and oatmeal is also rich in saponins and the hard-to-get GLA, an essential fatty acid.

Organic live yogurt. A good source a few times a week of beneficial bacteria for the digestive tract. Keeping the bacterial balance right will help keep the urinary tract free of infection. Eat only "live" yogurts made from the milk of organically reared animals to avoid encountering hormones, antibiotics and other chemicals added to animal feed.

Cranberry juice. Keeps bacteria from sticking to the urinary tract, so a daily glassful is a precautionary measure against infection if you have a tendency to get urinary tract infections. However, please don't drink the sugar-laden varieties.

Water, water, water! This is an essential, but often forgotten nutrient required for the processing of all the others. Dehydration stresses the prostate while about eight glasses of clean water a day will keep your system well supplied. Mild herb teas make a pleasant variation and a worthwhile switch from coffee, a prostate irritant.

HOW TO IRRITATE THE PROSTATE!

On top of poor foods, it's easy to give your prostate a hard time with other substances. The following are all likely to keep the prostate gland working hard and under pressure:

Beer. This and other alcohol sources stimulate the growth-triggering mechanisms in BPH.

Caffeine. Even decaffeinated coffee has enough irritants to prove harmful to an aging, sensitive prostate. Sodas are another common source of caffeine, and chocolate contains a little. Go very easy on all sources. Herb teas are a much healthier beverage than coffee, and since many, such as chamomile, are calming, they can help alleviate stress that also contributes to harmful prostate chemistry. Try some ginseng tea to perk you up and support your reproductive system at the same time.

Tobacco. Never good for you! Smoking and other tobacco habits bring all kinds of toxins into the body, from nicotine to cadmium. Studies show there may be a greater risk of developing prostate cancer if you smoke and at least one study has shown a definite risk if smokers are exposed to other sources of cadmium. (Occupations such as welding and electroplating can lead, over time, to high levels of cadmium exposure.)

Environmental toxins. These include contaminants such as pesticides, dioxins and heavy metals. Synthetic hormones, too, should be avoided by consuming only whole, organic foods. Most livestock are fed hormones for fattening and antibiotics for disease prevention. Residues of these substances are found in foods. Even plastic can linings and butter wrapping can contain traces of synthetic estrogens. Contaminants like these become concentrated in the prostate gland, where they can lead to BPH by increasing the conversion of testosterone. The large increase in the incidence of BPH in the last few decades may in part reflect an increasing effect of toxic chemicals on human health.

References and Sources

Chaitow, L., *Prostate Troubles*, Thorsons, Harper Collins, London, 1988.

Challem, J., "Dietary Changes Can Protect Against Prostate Problems," *Let's Live*, July 1994:14-15, 18-20.

Donsbach, K., "Benign Prostatic Hypertrophy & Prostate Cancer," Rockland Corporation, 1994.

Gelbard, M., *Solving Prostate Problems*, Fireside, Simon & Schuster, New York, 1995.

Green, J., *The Male Herbal*, The Crossing Press, California, 1991.

Laing, C., "Abdominal Obesity Linked to BPH," *Medical Tribune*, Jan. 1, 1993.

Lipkin, R., "Vegemania—Scientists tout the health benefits of saponins," *Science News*, Dec. 9 1995:148:392-393.

Mabey, R., *The New Age Herbalist*, Collier Books, Macmillan Publishing, New York, 1988.

Murray, M. et al, *Encyclopedia of Natural Medicine*, Prima Publishing, 1991.

Murray, M., *Male Sexual Vitality*, Prima Publishing, 1994.

Murray, M., *The Healing Power of Herbs*, Prima Publishing, 1995.

Murray, M., *The Saw Palmetto Story*, Vital Communications, Washington, 1990.

Rosenbaum, A., "To Each His Own—Gentle herbal remedies for men," *Vegetarian Times*, Feb. 1993:186:75(5).

Steinman, D., "Enlarged Prostate? Try Tree Bark," *Natural Health*, July/Aug. 1994: 44-46.

Steinman, D., "Treating Prostate Troubles," *Natural Health*, Nov./Dec. 1993:56-59.

Stenson, J., "Prostate Cancer—Aggressive treatment unneeded for patients with low-grade tumors," *Medical Tribune*, Sept. 21, 1995:15.

Walsh, P., et al, *The Prostate*, Johns Hopkins University Press, 1995.

Weil, A., *Natural Health, Natural Medicine*, Houghton Mifflin, Boston, 1995.

INDEX

Dr. Earl Mindell's

What You Should Know About . . .
series
in print or forthcoming